Keto Diet Cookbook

Beginners

A Beginners Guide with Gorgeous

Keto Recipes for Burn Fat Fast on a

Budget

Matthew Buckley

Table of Contents

This declaration is deemed fair and valid by both the American Bar Association and the Committee of Publishers Association and is legally binding throughout the United States.

Furthermore, the transmission, duplication, or reproduction of any of the following work including specific information will be considered an illegal act irrespective of if it is done electronically or in print. This extends to creating a secondary or tertiary copy of the work or a recorded copy and is only allowed with the express written consent from the Publisher. All additional right reserved.

The information in the following pages is broadly considered a truthful and accurate account of facts and as such, any inattention, use, or misuse of the information in question by the reader will render any resulting actions solely under their purview. There are no scenarios in which the publisher or the original author of this work can be in any fashion deemed liable for any hardship or damages that may befall them after undertaking information described herein. Additionally, the information in the following pages is intended only for informational purposes and should thus be thought of as universal. As befitting its nature, it is presented without assurance regarding its prolonged validity or interim quality.

Trademarks that are mentioned are done without written consent and can in no way be considered an endorsement from the trademark holder.

INTRODUCTION

So the Ketogenic Diet is all about reducing the amount of carbohydrates you eat. Does this mean you won't get the kind of energy you need for the day? Of course not! It only means that now, your body has to find other possible sources of energy. Do you know where they will be getting that energy?

Even before we talk about how to do keto – it's important to first consider why this particular diet works. What actually happens to your body to make you lose weight?

As you probably know, the body uses food as an energy source. Everything you eat is turned into energy, so that you can get up and do whatever you need to accomplish for the day. The main energy source is sugar so what happens is that you eat something, the body breaks it down into sugar, and the sugar is processed into energy. Typically, the "sugar" is taken directly from the food you eat so if you eat just the right amount of food, then your body is fueled for the whole day. If you eat too much, then the sugar is stored in your body – hence the accumulation of fat.

But what happens if you eat less food? This is where the Ketogenic Diet comes in. You see, the process of creating sugar from food is usually faster if the food happens to be rich in carbohydrates. Bread, rice, grain, pasta – all of these are carbohydrates and they're the easiest food types to turn into energy. So here's the situation – you are eating less carbohydrates every day. To keep you energetic, the body breaks down the stored fat and turns them into molecules called ketone bodies. The process of turning the fat into ketone bodies is called "Ketosis" and obviously – this is where the name of the Ketogenic Diet comes from. The ketone bodies take the place of glucose in keeping you energetic. As long as you keep your carbohydrates reduced, the body will keep getting its energy from your body fat.

The Ketogenic Diet is often praised for its simplicity and when you look at it properly, the process is really straightforward. The Science behind the effectivity of the diet is also well-documented, and has been proven multiple times by different medical fields. For example, an article on Diet Review by Harvard provided a lengthy discussion on how the Ketogenic Diet works and why it is so effective for those who choose to use this diet.

But Fat Is the Enemy...Or Is It?

No – fat is NOT the enemy. Unfortunately, years of bad science told us that fat is something you have to avoid – but it's actually a very helpful thing for weight loss! Even before we move forward with this book, we'll have to discuss exactly what "healthy fats" are, and why they're actually the good guys. To do this, we need to make a distinction between the different kinds of fat. You've probably heard of them before and it is a little bit confusing at first. We'll try to go through them as simply as possible: Saturated fat. This is the kind you want to avoid. They're also called "solid fat" because each molecule is packed with hydrogen atoms. Simply put, it's the kind of fat that can easily cause a blockage in your body. It can raise cholesterol levels and lead to heart problems or a stroke. Saturated fat is something you can find in meat, dairy products, and other processed food items. Now, you're probably wondering: isn't the Ketogenic Diet packed with saturated fat? The answer is: not necessarily. You'll find later in the recipes given that the Ketogenic Diet promotes primarily unsaturated fat or healthy fat. While there are definitely many meat recipes in the list, most of these recipes contain healthy fat sources. Unsaturated Fat. These are the ones dubbed as healthy fat. They're the kind of fat you find in avocado, nuts, and other ingredients you usually find in Keto-friendly recipes. They're known to lower blood cholesterol and actually come in two types: polyunsaturated and monounsaturated. Both are good for your body but the benefits slightly vary, depending on what you're consuming.

Mushroom Omelet

Preparation Time: 5minutes

Cooking Time: 10minutes

Servings: 1

Ingredients:

- 4 sliced large mushrooms
- A quarter chopped yellow onion
- A single ounce of shredded cheese
- An ounce of butter
- 3 eggs

Directions:

1. Crack the eggs and whisk them.

2. When smooth and frothy, they are good.

3. Melt butter over medium heat in a frying pan.

4. Add onions and mushrooms and stir until they become tender.

5. Pour the egg mix in. Surround the veggies.

6. When the omelet begins to get firm but is still a little raw on top, add cheese.

7. Carefully ease around the edges and fold in half.

8. When it's golden brown underneath (turning this color), remove and plate it.

Nutrition: Calories: 517g Protein: 26g Fat: 4g Carbs: 5g

Crab Melt

Preparation Time: 5 minutes

Cooking Time: 20 minutes

Servings: 4

Ingredients:

- 2 zucchinis

- A single tablespoon olive oil

- 3 ounces of stalks from celery

- 3/4 cup of mayo

- 12 ounces of crab meat

- A single red bell pepper

- 7 ounces of cheese (use shredded cheddar)

- A single tablespoon of Dijon mustard

Direction:

1. Preheat your oven to 450.

2. Slice your zucchini lengthwise. Go for about a half-inch thick.

3. Add salt.

4. Let it sit for 15 minutes.

5. Pat it dries with a paper towel.

6. Place your slices on a baking sheet.

7. The baking sheet needs to be lined with parchment paper.

8. Brush olive oil on each side.

9. Finely chop the vegetables.

10.   Mix with the other ingredients.

11.   Apply mix to zucchini.

12.   Bake for 20 minutes. Your top will be golden brown.

Nutrition: Calories-742 Fat-65 grams Fiber-3 grams Carbs-7 grams Protein-30 grams

Poblano Peppers

Preparation Time: 5minutes

Cooking Time: 15minutes

Servings: 2

Ingredients

- A pound of grated cauliflower

- 3 ounces of butter

- 4 eggs

- 3 ounces of poblano peppers

- A single tablespoon of olive oil

- Half a cup of mayo

Directions:

1. Put your mayo in a bowl to the side.

2. Grate the cauliflower, including the stem.

3. Fry the cauliflower for 5 minutes in the butter.

4. Brush the oil on the peppers.

5. Fry them until you see the skin bubble a

   little.

6. Fry your eggs any way you like.

7. Serve with mayo.

Nutrition:

Calories: 898

Fat: 87g

Protein: 17g

Carbs: 9g

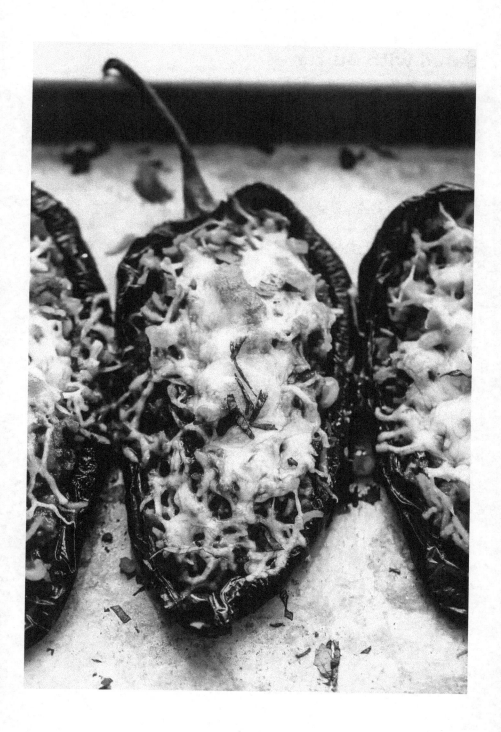

Salad with Butter

Preparation Time: 5minutes

Cooking Time: 10minutes

Servings: 2

Ingredients:

- 10 ounces of goat cheese

- A quarter cup of pumpkin seeds

- 2 ounces of butter

- Tablespoons of balsamic vinegar

- 3 ounces of spinach (use baby spinach)

Directions:

1. Preheat oven to 400.

2. Put goat cheese in a baking dish that is greased.

3. Bake 10 minutes.

4. Toast pumpkin seeds in a frying pan that is dry. The temperature should be fairly high. They need some color, and they should start to pop.

5. Lower heat.

6. Add butter and simmer till it smells nutty and is golden brown.

7. Add vinegar and boil 3 minutes.

8. Turn off heat.

9. Spread the spinach on your plate and top with cheese and sauce.

Nutrition: Calories: 824 Fat: 73g Protein: 37g Carbs: 3g

Tuna Casserole

Preparation Time 7minutes

Cooking Time 20minutes

Serving: 4

Ingredients:

- A single green bell pepper

- 5 ⅓ celery stalks

- 16 ounces of tuna in olive oil and drained

- A single yellow onion

- 2 ounces of butter

- A single cup of mayo

- 4 ounces of parmesan cheese freshly shredded

- A single teaspoon of chili flakes

Directions:

1. Preheat your oven to 400.

2. Chop all of the bell peppers, onions, and celery finely before frying it in butter in a frying pan. They should be slightly soft.

3. Mix mayo and tuna with the flakes and cheese.

4. This should be done in a greased baking dish.

5. Add the veggies.

6. Stir.

7. Bake 20 minutes.

8. It should be golden brown.

Nutrition:

Calories: 953

Fat: 83g

Protein: 43g

Carbs: 5g

Goat Cheese Frittata

Preparation Time: 15minutes

Cooking Time: 30minutes

Servings: 2

Ingredients:

- 4 ounces of goat cheese

- 5 ounces of mushrooms

- 3 ounces of fresh spinach

- 2 ounces of scallions

- 2 ounces of butter

- Half a dozen eggs

Directions:

1. Preheat your oven to 350.

2. Crack the eggs and whisk before crumbling cheese in the mix.

3. Cut mushrooms into wedge shapes.

4. Chop up the scallions.

5. Melt the butter in a skillet that is oven proof and cook scallions and mushrooms over medium heat for 10 minutes. They will be golden brown (or should be).

6. Add spinach and sauté two minutes.

7. Pour egg mixture into the skillet.

8. Place in the oven uncovered and bake 20 minutes.

9. It should be golden brown in the center.

Nutrition:

Calories: 774

Fat: 67g

Carbs: 6g

Protein: 35g

Pancakes

Preparation Time: 5 minutes

Cooking Time: 6 minutes

Servings: 2

Ingredients

- ¼ cup almond flour
- 1 ½ tbsp. unsalted butter
- 2 oz. cream cheese, softened
- 2 eggs

Directions:

1. Take a bowl, crack eggs in it, whisk well until fluffy, and then whisk in flour and cream cheese until well combined.

2. Take a skillet pan, place it over medium heat, add butter and when it melts, drop pancake batter in four sections, spread it

evenly, and cook for 2 minutes per side until brown.

3. Serve.

Nutrition:

166.8 Calories;

15 g Fats;

5.8 g Protein;

1.8 g Net Carb;

0.8 g Fiber;

Cheese Roll-Ups

Preparation Time: 5 minutes

Cooking Time: 0 minutes

Servings: 2

Ingredients

- 2 oz. mozzarella cheese, sliced, full-fat

- 1-ounce butter, unsalted

Directions:

1. Cut cheese into slices and then cut butter into thin slices.

2. Top each cheese slice with a slice of butter, roll it and then serve.

Nutrition:

166 Calories; 15 g

Fats; 6.5 g

Protein; 2 g

Net Carb; 0 g

Fiber;

Scrambled Eggs with Spinach and Cheese

Preparation Time: 5 minutes

Cooking Time: 5 minutes

Servings: 2

Ingredients

- 2 oz. spinach

- 2 eggs

- 1 tbsp. coconut oil

- 2 tbsp. grated mozzarella cheese, full-fat

- Seasoning:

- ¼ tsp salt

- 1/8 tsp ground black pepper

- 1/8 tsp red pepper flakes

Directions:

1. Take a medium bowl, crack eggs in it, add salt and black pepper and whisk until combined.

2. Take a medium skillet pan, place it over medium heat, add oil and when hot, add spinach and cook for 1 minute until leaves wilt.

3. Pour eggs over spinach, stir and cook for 1 minute until just set.

4. Stir in cheese, then remove the pan from heat and sprinkle red pepper flakes on top.

5. Serve.

Nutrition: 171 Calories; 14 g Fats; 9.2 g Protein; 1.1 g Net Carb; 1.7 g Fiber;

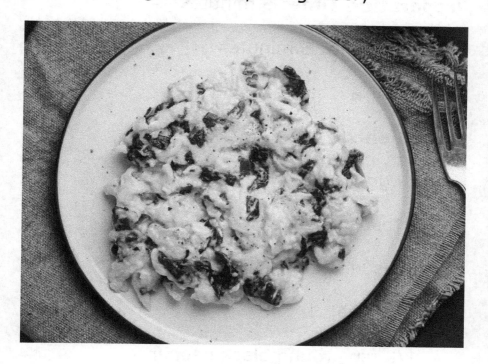

Egg Wraps

Preparation Time: 5 minutes

Cooking Time: 5 minutes

Servings: 2

Ingredients

- 2 eggs

- 1 tbsp. coconut oil

- Seasoning:

- ¼ tsp salt

- 1/8 tsp ground black pepper

Directions:

Take a medium bowl, crack eggs in it, add salt and black pepper, and then whisk until blended.

Take a frying pan, place it over medium-low heat, add coconut oil and when it melts, pour in half of the egg, spread it evenly into a thin layer by rotating the pan and cook for 2 minutes.

Then flip the pan, cook for 1 minute, and transfer to a plate.

Repeat with the remaining egg to make another wrap, then roll each egg wrap and serve.

Nutrition: 68 Calories; 4.7 g Fats; 5.5 g Protein; 0.5 g Net Carb; 0 g Fiber;

Chaffles with Poached Eggs

Preparation Time: 5 minutes

Cooking Time: 10 minutes

Servings: 2

Ingredients

- 2 tsp coconut flour
- ½ cup shredded cheddar cheese, full-fat
- 3 eggs
- Seasoning:
- ¼ tsp salt
- 1/8 tsp ground black pepper

Directions:

1. Switch on a mini waffle maker and let it preheat for 5 minutes.

2. Meanwhile, take a medium bowl, place all the ingredients in it, reserving 2 eggs and then mix by using an immersion blender until smooth.

3. Ladle the batter evenly into the waffle maker, shut with lid, and let it cook for 3 to 4 minutes until firm and golden brown.

4. Meanwhile, prepare poached eggs, and for this, take a medium bowl half full with water, place it over medium heat and bring it to a boil.

5. Then crack an egg in a ramekin, carefully pour it into the boiling water and cook for 3 minutes.

6. Transfer egg to a plate lined with paper towels by using a slotted spoon and repeat with the other egg.

7. Top chaffles with poached eggs, season with salt and black pepper, and then serve.

Nutrition:

265 Calories; 18.5 g

Fats; 17.6 g

Protein;

3.4 g Net

Carb; 6 g Fiber;

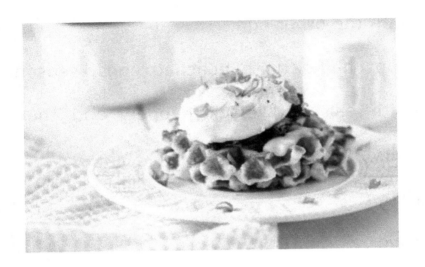

Chaffle with Scrambled Eggs

Preparation Time: 5 minutes

Cooking Time: 10 minutes

Servings: 2

Ingredients

- 2 tsp coconut flour

- ½ cup shredded cheddar cheese, full-fat

- 3 eggs

- 1-ounce butter, unsalted

- Seasoning:

- ¼ tsp salt

- 1/8 tsp ground black pepper

- 1/8 tsp dried oregano

Directions:

1. Switch on a mini waffle maker and let it preheat for 5 minutes.

2. Meanwhile, take a medium bowl, place all the ingredients in it, reserving 2 eggs and then mix by using an immersion blender until smooth.

3. Ladle the batter evenly into the waffle maker, shut with lid, and let it cook for 3 to 4 minutes until firm and golden brown.

4. Meanwhile, prepare scrambled eggs and for this, take a medium bowl, crack the eggs in it and whisk them with a fork until frothy, and then season with salt and black pepper.

5. Take a medium skillet pan, place it over medium heat, add butter and when it melts, pour in eggs and cook for 2 minutes until creamy, stirring continuously.

6. Top chaffles with scrambled eggs, sprinkle with oregano, and then serve.

Nutrition:

265 Calories;

18.5 g Fats;

17.6 g Protein;

3.4 g Net Carb;

6 g Fiber;

Sheet Pan Eggs with Mushrooms and Spinach

Preparation Time: 5 minutes

Cooking Time: 12 minutes

Servings: 2

Ingredients

- 2 eggs

- 1 tsp chopped jalapeno pepper

- 1 tbsp. chopped mushrooms

- 1 tbsp. chopped spinach

- 1 tbsp. chopped chard

- Seasoning:

- 1/3 tsp salt

- 1/4 tsp ground black pepper

Directions:

1. Turn on the oven, then set it to 350 degrees F and let it preheat.

2. Take a medium bowl, crack eggs in it, add salt and black pepper, then add all the vegetables and stir until combined.

3. Take a medium sheet ball or rimmed baking sheet, grease it with oil, pour prepared egg batter on it, and then bake for 10 to 12 minutes until done.

4. Cut egg into two squares and then serve.

Nutrition: 165 Calories; 10.7 g Fats; 14 g Protein; 1.5 g Net Carb; 0.5 g Fiber;

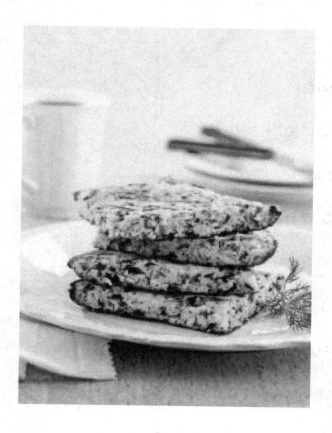

No Bread Breakfast Sandwich

Preparation Time: 10 minutes

Cooking Time: 15 minutes

Servings: 2

Ingredients

- 2 slices of ham

- 4 eggs

- 1 tsp tabasco sauce

- 3 tbsp. butter, unsalted

- 2 tsp grated mozzarella cheese

- Seasoning:

- ¼ tsp salt

- 1/8 tsp ground black pepper

Directions:

1. Take a frying pan, place it over medium

   heat, add butter and when it melt, crack

an egg in it and fry for 2 to 3 minutes until cooked to desired level.

2. Transfer fried egg to a plate, fry remaining eggs in the same manner and when done, season eggs with salt and black pepper.

3. Prepare the sandwich and for this, use a fried egg as a base for sandwich, then top with a ham slice, sprinkle with a tsp of ham and cover with another fried egg.

4. Place egg into the pan, return it over low heat and let it cook until cheese melts.

5. Prepare another sandwich in the same manner and then serve.

Nutrition:

180 Calories; 15 g

Fats; 10 g

Protein; 1 g

Net Carb; 0 g

Fiber;

Scrambled Eggs with Basil and Butter

Preparation Time: 5 minutes

Cooking Time: 5 minutes

Servings: 2

Ingredients

- 1 tbsp. chopped basil leaves

- 2 tbsp. butter, unsalted

- 2 tbsp. grated cheddar cheese

- 2 eggs

- 2 tbsp. whipping cream

- Seasoning:

- 1/8 tsp salt

- 1/8 tsp ground black pepper

Directions:

1. Take a medium bowl, crack eggs in it, add salt, black pepper, cheese and cream and whisk until combined.

2. Take a medium pan, place it over low heat, add butter and when it melts, pour in the egg mixture and cook for 2 to 3 minutes until eggs have scrambled to the desired level.

3. When done, distribute scrambled eggs between two plates, top with basil leaves and then serve.

Nutrition: 320 Calories; 29 g Fats; 13 g Protein; 1.5 g Net Carb; 0 g Fiber;

Bacon and Eggs

Preparation Time: 5 minutes

Cooking Time: 10 minutes

Servings: 2

Ingredients

- 2 eggs

- 4 slices of turkey bacon

- ¼ tsp salt

- ¼ tsp ground black pepper

Directions:

1. Take a skillet pan, place it over medium heat, add bacon slices in it and cook for 5 minutes until crispy.

2. Transfer bacon slices to a plate and set aside until required, reserving the fat in the pan.

3. Cook the egg in the pan one at a time, and for this, crack an egg in the pan and cook for 2 to 3 minutes or more until the egg has cooked to desire level.

4. Transfer egg to a plate and cook the other egg in the same manner.

5. Season eggs with salt and black pepper and then serve with cooked bacon.

Nutrition:

136 Calories;

11 g Fats;

7.5 g Protein;

1 g Net Carb;

0 g Fiber

Boiled Eggs

Preparation Time: 5 minutes

Cooking Time: 10 minutes

Servings: 2

Ingredients

- 2 eggs

- ½ of a medium avocado

- Seasoning:

- ¼ tsp salt

- ¼ tsp ground black pepper

Directions:

1. Place a medium pot over medium heat, fill it half full with water and bring it to boil.

2. Then carefully place the eggs in the boiling water and boil the eggs for 5 minutes until

soft-boiled, 8 minutes for medium-boiled, and 10 minutes for hard-boiled.

3. When eggs have boiled, transfer them to a bowl containing chilled water and let them rest for 5 minutes.

4. Then crack the eggs with a spoon and peel them.

5. Cut each egg into slices, season with salt and black pepper, and serve with diced avocado.

Nutrition: 112 Calories; 9.5 g Fats; 5.5 g Protein; 1 g Net Carb; 0 g Fiber;

Spicy Cheese Chicken Soup

Preparation Time: 15 MINUTES

Cooking Time: 40 MINUTES

Servings: 4

Ingredients

- ½ cup salsa enchilada verde

- 2 cups chicken, cooked and shredded

- 2 cups chicken or bone broth

- 1 cup cheddar cheese, shredded

- 4 ounces cream cheese

- ½ tsp chili powder

- ½ tsp cumin, ground

- ½ tsp fresh cilantro, chopped

- Salt and black pepper to taste

Directions

1. Combine the cream cheese, salsa verde, and broth in a food processor.

2. Pulse until smooth. Transfer the mixture to a pot and place over medium heat.

3. Cook until hot, but do not bring to a boil.

4. Add chicken, chili powder, and cumin, and cook for about 3-5 minutes, or until it is heated through. Stir in Cheddar cheese. Season with salt and pepper to taste.

5. Serve hot in individual bowls sprinkled with fresh cilantro.

Nutrition Calories 346, Net Carbs 3g, Fat 23g,

Protein 25g

Cheese & Spinach Stuffed Chicken

Preparation Time: 50 MINUTES

Cooking Time: 40 MINUTES

Servings: 4

Ingredients

- 4 chicken breasts, boneless and skinless

- ½ cup mozzarella cheese

- 1 ½ cups Parmesan cheese, shredded

- 6 ounces cream cheese

- 2 cups spinach, chopped

- A pinch of nutmeg

- ½ tsp garlic, minced

- <u>Breading</u>

- 2 eggs, beaten

- 1/3 cup almond flour

- 2 tbsp. olive oil

- ½ tsp parsley

- 1/3 cup Parmesan cheese

- A pinch of onion powder

Directions

1. Pound the chicken until it doubles in size. Mix cream cheese, spinach, mozzarella cheese, nutmeg, and salt, pepper, and Parmesan cheese in a bowl. Divide the mixture between the chicken breasts and spread it out evenly. Wrap the chicken in a plastic wrap. Refrigerate for 15 minutes.

2. Preheat the oven to 370 F.

3. Beat the eggs and set aside. Combine all of the other breading ingredients in a bowl. Dip the chicken in eggs first, then in the breading mixture.

4. Warm the olive oil in a pan over medium heat. Cook the chicken in the pan until browned, about 5-6 minutes. Place on a lined baking sheet, and bake for 20 minutes. Serve.

Nutrition

Calories 491,

Net Carbs 3.5g,

Fat 36g,

Protein 38g

Chicken & Spinach Gratin

Preparation Time: 45 MINUTES

Cooking Time: 40 MINUTES

Servings: 6

Ingredients

- 6 chicken breasts, skinless and boneless

- 1 tsp mixed spice seasoning

- Pink salt and black pepper to season

- 2 loose cups baby spinach

- 3 tsp olive oil

- 4 oz. cream cheese, cubed

- 1 ¼ cups mozzarella cheese, shredded

- 4 tbsp. water

Directions

1. Preheat oven to 375 F.

2. Season chicken with spice mix, salt, and black pepper. Pat with your hands to have the seasoning stick on the chicken.

3. Put in the casserole dish and layer spinach over the chicken.

4. Mix the oil with cream cheese, mozzarella, salt, and black pepper and stir in water a tablespoon at a time.

5. Pour the mixture over the chicken and cover the pot with aluminum foil.

6. Bake for 20 minutes, remove foil and continue cooking for 15 minutes until a beautiful golden brown color is formed on top.

7. Take out and allow sitting for 5 minutes.

Serve warm with braised asparagus.

Nutrition

Calories 340,

Net Carbs 1g,

Fat 30.2g,

Protein 15g

Weekend Chicken with Grapefruit & Lemon

Preparation Time: 30 MINUTES

Cooking Time: 40 MINUTES

Servings: 4

Ingredients

- 1 cup omission IPA
- A pinch of garlic powder
- 1 tsp grapefruit zest
- 3 tbsp. lemon juice
- ½ tsp coriander, ground
- 1 tbsp. fish sauce
- 2 tbsp. butter
- ¼ tsp xanthan gum
- 3 tbsp. swerve sweetener
- 20 chicken wing pieces

- Salt and black pepper to taste

Directions

1. Combine lemon juice and zest, fish sauce, coriander, omission IPA, sweetener, and garlic powder in a saucepan.

2. Bring to a boil, cover, lower the heat, and let simmer for 10 minutes.

3. Stir in the butter and xanthan gum. Set aside. Season the wings with some salt and pepper.

4. Preheat the grill and cook for 5 minutes per side.

5. Serve topped with the sauce.

Nutrition

Calories 365,

Net Carbs 4g,

Fat 25g,

Protein 21g

Bacon-Wrapped Chicken with Grilled Asparagus

Preparation Time: 50 MINUTES

Cooking Time: 40 MINUTES

Servings: 4

Ingredients

- 2 tbsp. fresh lemon juice

- 6 chicken breasts

- 8 bacon slices

- 1 tbsp. olive oil

- 1 lb. asparagus spears

- 3 tbsp. olive oil

- Salt and black pepper to taste

- Manchego cheese for topping

Directions

1. Preheat the oven to 400 F.

2. Season chicken breasts with salt and black pepper, and wrap 2 bacon slices around each chicken breast. Arrange on a baking sheet that is lined with parchment paper, drizzle with oil, and bake for 25-30 minutes until bacon is brown and crispy.

3. Preheat the grill.

4. Brush the asparagus spears with olive oil and season with salt. Grill turning frequently until slightly charred, 5-10 minutes.

5. Remove to a plate and drizzle with lemon juice. Grate over Manchego cheese so that

it melts a little on contact with the hot asparagus and forms a cheesy dressing.

Nutrition

Calories 468,

Net Carbs 2g,

Fat 38g,

Protein 26g

Bok Choy Caesar Salad with Chicken

PREPARATION TIME: 1 HOUR AND 20 MINUTES

COOKING TIME: 40 MINUTES

SERVINGS: 4

Ingredients

- <u>Chicken</u>
- 4 chicken thighs, boneless and skinless
- ¼ cup lemon juice
- 2 garlic cloves, minced
- 2 tbsp. olive oil
- <u>Salad</u>
- ½ cup caesar salad dressing, sugar-free
- 2 tbsp. olive oil
- 12 bok choy leaves
- 3 Parmesan cheese crisps

- Parmesan cheese, grated or garnishing

Directions

1. Combine the chicken ingredients in a Ziploc bag. Seal the bag, shake to combine, and refrigerate for 1 hour.

2. Preheat the grill to medium heat, and grill the chicken about 4 minutes per side.

3. Cut bok choy leaves lengthwise, and brush it with oil. Grill for about 3 minutes. Place on a serving platter. Top with the chicken, and drizzle the dressing over. Sprinkle with Parmesan cheese and finish with Parmesan crisps to serve.

Nutrition

Calories 529,

 Net Carbs 5g,

Fat 39g,

Protein 33g

Turkey Patties with Cucumber Salsa

Preparation Time: 30 MINUTES

Cooking Time: 40 MINUTES

Servings: 4

Ingredients

- 2 spring onions, thinly sliced

- 1 pound turkey, ground

- 1 egg

- 2 garlic cloves, minced

- 1 tbsp. herbs, chopped

- 1 small chili pepper, deseeded and diced

- 2 tbsp. ghee

- Cucumber Salsa:

- 1 tbsp. apple cider vinegar

- 1 tbsp. dill, chopped

- 1 garlic clove, minced

- 2 cucumbers, grated

- 1 cup sour cream

- 1 jalapeño pepper, minced

- 2 tbsp. olive oil

Directions

1. Place all of the turkey ingredients, except the ghee, in a bowl. Mix to combine. Make patties out of the mixture.

2. Melt ghee in a skillet over medium heat. Cook the patties for 3 minutes per side.

3. Place all of the salsa ingredients in a bowl and mix to combine. Serve the patties topped with salsa.

Nutrition Calories 475, Net Carbs 5g, Fat 38g,

Protein 26g

Chili Chicken Kabobs with Tahini Dressing

Preparation Time: 20 MINUTES+ 2 HOURS REFRIGERATION

Cooking Time: 10 MINUTES

Servings: 6

Ingredients

- 3 tbsp. soy sauce
- 1 tbsp. ginger-garlic paste
- 2 tbsp. swerve brown sugar
- 2 tbsp. olive oil
- 3 chicken breasts, cut into bite-sized cubes
- ½ cup tahini
- ½ tsp garlic powder
- Salt and chili pepper to taste

Directions

1. In a bowl, whisk soy sauce, ginger-garlic paste, swerve brown sugar, chili pepper, and olive oil. Put the chicken in a zipper bag, pour the marinade over, seal, and shake for an even coat. Marinate in the fridge for 2 hours.

2. Preheat a grill to 400 F and thread the chicken on skewers. Cook for 10 minutes in total with three to four turnings to be golden brown. Plate them.

3. Mix the tahini, garlic powder, salt, and ¼ cup of warm water in a bowl. Serve the chicken skewers and tahini dressing with cauliflower fried rice.

Nutrition Calories 225, Net Carbs 2g, Fat 17.4g, Protein 15g

Strawberry Buckwheat Pancakes

Preparation Time: 20 minutes

Cooking Time: 5 minutes

Servings: 4

Ingredients:

- 100g (3½oz) strawberries, chopped

- 100g (3½ oz.) buckwheat flour

- 1 egg

- 250mls (8fl oz.) milk

- 1 teaspoon olive oil

- 1 teaspoon olive oil for frying

- Freshly squeezed juice of 1 orange

- 175 calories per serving

Directions:

1. Pour the milk into a bowl and mix in the egg and a teaspoon of olive oil. Sift in the flour to the liquid mixture until smooth and creamy. Allow it to rest for 15 minutes. Heat a little oil in a pan and pour in a quarter of the mixture (or to the size you prefer.) Sprinkle in a quarter of the strawberries into the batter. Cook for around 2 minutes on each side. Serve hot with a drizzle of orange juice. You could try experimenting with other berries such as blueberries and blackberries

Nutrition: Calories Fat Fiber Carbs Protein

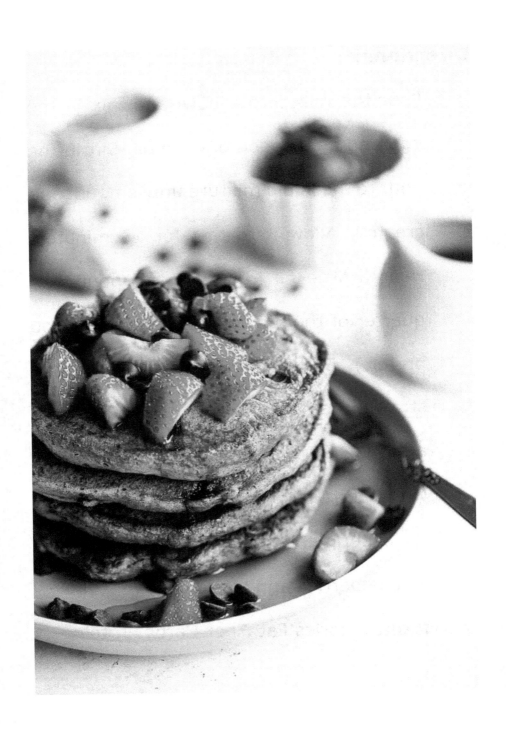

Strawberry & Nut Granola

Preparation Time: 10 minutes

Cooking Time: 50 minutes

Servings: 12

Ingredients:

- 200g (7oz) oats
- 250g (9oz) buckwheat flakes
- 100g (3½ oz.) walnuts, chopped
- 100g (3½ oz.) almonds, chopped
- 100g (3½ oz.) dried strawberries
- 1½ teaspoons ground ginger
- 1½ teaspoons ground cinnamon
- 120mls (4fl oz.) olive oil
- 2 tablespoon honey

Directions:

1. Combine the oats, buckwheat flakes, nuts, ginger and cinnamon. In a saucepan, warm the oil and honey. Stir until the honey has melted. Pour the warm oil into the dry ingredients and mix well. Spread the mixture out on a large baking tray (or two) and bake in the oven at 150C (300F) for around 50 minutes until the granola is golden. Allow it to cool. Add in the dried berries. Store in an airtight container until ready to use. Can be served with yogurt, milk or even dry as a handy snack.

Nutrition:

Calories 391 Fat 0 Fiber 6 Carbs 3 Protein 8

Chilled Strawberry & Walnut Porridge

Preparation Time: 10 minutes

Cooking Time: 0 minutes

Servings: 1

Ingredients:

- 100g (3½ oz.) strawberries

- 50g (2oz) rolled oats

- 4 walnut halves, chopped

- 1 teaspoon chia seeds

- 200mls (7fl oz.) unsweetened soya milk

- 100ml (3½ FL oz.) water

Directions:

1. Place the strawberries, oats, soya milk and water into a blender and process until smooth. Stir in the chia seeds and mix well. Chill in the fridge overnight and serve

in the morning with a sprinkling of chopped walnuts. It's simple and delicious.

Nutrition:

Calories 384 Fat 2 Fiber 5 Carbs 3 Protein7

Fruit & Nut Yogurt Crunch

Preparation Time: 5 minutes

Cooking Time: 0 minutes

Servings: 1

Ingredients:

- 100g (3½ oz.) plain Greek yogurt

- 50g (2oz) strawberries, chopped

- 6 walnut halves, chopped

- Sprinkling of cocoa powder

Directions:

1. Stir half of the chopped strawberries into the yogurt. Using a glass, place a layer of yogurt with a sprinkling of strawberries and walnuts, followed by another layer of the same until you reach the top of the

glass. Garnish with walnuts pieces and a dusting of cocoa powder.

Nutrition:

Calories 296 Fat 4 Fiber 2 Carbs 5 Protein 9

Cheesy Baked Eggs

Preparation Time: 5 minutes

Cooking Time: 15 minutes

Servings: 4

Ingredients:

- 4 large eggs

- 75g (3oz) cheese, grated

- 25g (1oz) fresh rocket (arugula) leaves, finely chopped

- 1 tablespoon parsley

- ½ teaspoon ground turmeric

- 1 tablespoon olive oil

Directions:

1. Grease each ramekin dish with a little olive oil. Divide the rocket (arugula) between the ramekin dishes then break an egg into

each one. Sprinkle a little parsley and turmeric on top then sprinkle on the cheese. Place the ramekins in a preheated oven at 220C/425F for 15 minutes, until the eggs are set and the cheese is bubbling.

Nutrition: Calories 198 Fat 9 Fiber 3 Carbs 2 Protein 13

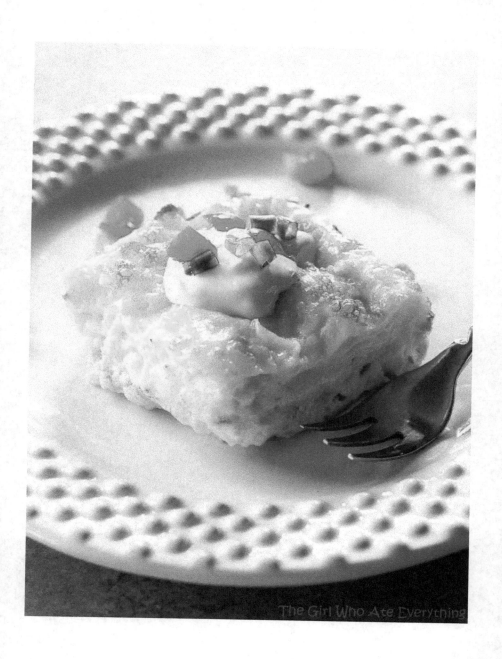

CONCLUSION

The things to watch out for when coming off keto are weight gain, bloating, more energy, and feeling hungry. The weight gain is nothing to freak out over; perhaps, you might not even gain any. It all depends on your diet, how your body processes carbs, and, of course, water weight. The length of your keto diet is a significant factor in how much weight you have lost, which is caused by the reduction of carbs. The bloating will occur because of the reintroduction of fibrous foods and your body getting used to digesting them again. The bloating van lasts for a few days to a few weeks. You will feel like you have more energy because carbs break down into glucose, which is the body's primary source of fuel. You may also notice better brain function and the ability to work out more.

Whether you have met your weight loss goals, your life changes, or you simply want to eat whatever you want again. You cannot just suddenly start consuming carbs again for it will shock your system. Have an idea of what you want to allow back into your consumption slowly. Be familiar with portion sizes and stick to that amount of carbs for the first few times you eat post-keto. Start with non-processed carbs like whole grain, beans, and fruits. Start slow and see how your body responds before resolving to add carbs one meal at a time.

The ketogenic diet is the ultimate tool you can use to plan your future. Can you picture being more involved, more productive and efficient, and more relaxed and energetic? That future is possible for you, and it does not have to be a complicated process to achieve that vision. You can choose right now to be healthier and slimmer and more fulfilled tomorrow. It is possible with the ketogenic diet. It does not just improve your physical health but your mental and emotional health as well. This diet improves your health holistically. Do not give up now as there will be quite a few days where you may think to yourself, "Why am I doing this?" and to answer that, simply focus on the goals you wish to achieve. A good diet enriched with all the proper nutrients is our best shot of achieving an active metabolism and efficient lifestyle. A lot of people think that the Keto diet is simply for people who are interested in losing weight. You will find that it is quite the opposite. There are intense keto diets where only 5 percent of the diet comes from carbs, 20 percent is from protein, and 75 percent is from fat. But even a modified version of this which involves consciously choosing foods low in carbohydrate and high in healthy fats is good enough. Thanks for reading this book. I hope it has provided you with enough insight to get you going. Don't put off getting started. The sooner you begin this diet, the sooner you'll start to notice an improvement in your health and well-being.

CPSIA information can be obtained
at www.ICGtesting.com
Printed in the USA
BVHW091923230621
610293BV00007B/753

9 781803 041469